Caregiver Important Information

Being Proactive - "Don't Wait For A Problem"

Michelle Bever

Please remember to leave a review if this information has helped you, a family member, and/or someone you know as it is greatly appreciated!

Thank you!

Copyright © 2021, Michelle Bever

All rights reserved. No part of this book may be reproduced, stored, or transmitted by any means—whether auditory, graphic, mechanical, or electronic—without written permission of both publisher and author, except in the case of brief excerpts used in critical articles and reviews. Unauthorized reproduction of any part of this work is illegal and is punishable by law.

Table Of Contents

Special Thanks.. 1
Our Story.. 2
Doctors... 7
Sugar and Salt.. 10
Documentation... 11
Tests... 13
Eyes Open.. 15
Communication.. 18
Stages... 19
Home Care... 21
Your List... 22

Special Thanks

A goal cannot be achieved without the special interaction of people who genuinely care about you, what you are doing, and how it can help others. Without faith and determination I would not be able to finish my books and get them published online and I give thanks to the Lord most of all.

My mother and father had faith in my abilities to look for solutions and helped give me the fortitude to seek solutions. I will be forever grateful to them for this.

Thank you to all the CNA's, Nurses, and Doctors who have worked with me to provide the best care for my mother.

Linda, my sister-in-law, has shared information that has been very helpful in making my mother's life better.

My husband, Brian, who has been so incredibly supportive and I would not have been able to do any of this without him. He stood with me through it all and that is priceless.

Our Story

Our story starts with my father passing away, and my mother, who had been good about taking her medications, decided that she did not need to take them regularly anymore. My mother has always had a depression problem that I did not know about until becoming an adult. She did pretty well for a while without anyone noticing but within time, pills were found on the floor by family members.

Mom not taking her pills brought about a concern, but of course, my mother downplayed it and said she was an adult who could take care of herself.

My mother later got into a few accidents and fortunately no one got hurt but this further concerned our family. When mom kept forgetting her pills she stopped going places, getting groceries, and taking care of herself.

I lived out of state, and fortunately, my mother's friends stopped by and brought her food. A family member took advantage of this situation and got themselves placed a power of attorney. Initially, we thought they were helping mom but found out that they were only helping themselves to my mother's money by continually draining it. This person would take money every time they went to the store and even got into her cd accounts, cashing almost all of them before being caught.

I flew out and took over my mother's accounts after this family member chose to flee to another state to avoid being prosecuted. My father had been a veteran, and benefits that would have paid for my mother's prescriptions in full were not utilized, leaving a mess to clean up in a multitude of ways.

My husband and I had to move my mother to where we live to ensure that we could take care of her correctly. While my mother still had her faculties, we had a trust made to speak for her when she could not speak for herself anymore. She was happy to know her specific wishes would be listened to.

Mom was doing better since now, with her prescriptions regulated, I could find a senior home close to my home. Mom was happy as it was a very beautiful place, and I would set up all her prescriptions. I would call to make sure she would take her prescriptions on time or show up. She seemed to be doing better and even took the bus to get groceries, do laundry, and sometimes meet up with the other ladies for the dinners inside where she lived.

Within a year, mom started to act out about me checking to see if she had taken her prescriptions stating she was an adult who had taken care of herself for a long time. I never knew if I would be seeing a nice mother or a mean one. I took her to all her doctor's appointments, and each time they said she was fine. As her moods worsened, I asked the doctor whether she needed to increase or decrease her medication, but they just said she was fine. I am not a doctor, so I did not question as I do now.

Mom started to get worse again and became verbally abusive and mean at times. The final straw was when she lied to me about taking her prescriptions, and I came into her apartment with mom on the bathroom floor with only a top on. She had double dosed since she was forgetting and also did not want me to know.

I called 911, and then the paramedics came to check her out to make sure she was okay. They took mom to the hospital, which gave me time to see what state-funded assisted living facilities were available. I was blessed to find one that I liked what I saw, and they had a one-bedroom that just had to be cleaned. After filling out the papers, I immediately put down the down payment for the one bedroom. The additional blessing was that there was a rehabilitation and nursing facility right across the street.

Mom moved into her new one-bedroom in the assisted living, and it was great as they gave the prescriptions on a schedule and regularly checked each person. It was also close to my home, so I could see her and spend time with her.

The prescriptions mom was taking were the same and then later continued to affect her. Mom fell twice while in the assisted living facility, and the last one fractured her spine. This was while being monitored and taking prescriptions regularly. My mother's attitude was also up and down.

When mom went into the hospital the last time for a fractured spine, they initially sent her back home. I went to the hospital and advocated for her till they admitted her as the pain was too much. While admitted, a doctor blessed my mother by looking over all of my mother's medications. This doctor canceled some prescriptions, halved others, and only left a few full. They were her thyroid, high blood pressure, and depression medication.

My mother was then brought over to the rehab facility to recover, and while there, she still was having problems with the medications. Again, I wondered what should we do? Do we increase, decrease, add another as sometimes they do to balance? When the doctor decreased the medications and canceled others, a lot of questions arose.

The rehab and nursing facility doctor worked with me to figure out what my mother may need. This led to my mother feeling like she was on a cruise boat and wondering when she would be back on land. She could not remember and felt scared since she felt off; even though she was much nicer to me, it was not worth what she was going through. I had those stopped immediately, and then we were back at square one. My mother also had stopped wanting to eat, which was scary. We needed to find out what could help my mother, and it was time to learn from the doctor who had made changes earlier. There had been a reason for that, and so I looked at all the prescriptions for a closer look.

My sister-in-law, Linda, helped bring attention to the many confusions about medications and tests to see what is right for the person. She had been a caregiver to some of her relatives and had learned from those experiences. Her love for my brother and want to help answer some of my questions led us to become a formidable team.

I looked up the depression medication that my mother was on and looked up the symptoms of being over-medicated. My mother had almost all of them. I researched and printed out all of this information. I typed up a letter addressing what I had found and detailed information supporting my request to decrease her depression medication.

Where my mother is, the staff has always been available to listen to any concerns I have about my mom. After reading my letter and looking at my documentation, the doctor on staff agreed to decrease her prescription. Within a week, my mother was more alert, ate more, and was nicer. Eventually, my mother was taken off her depression medication over the next few years, and we have a very loving relationship. I am so thankful she is okay and that I can spend quality time with her.

Our story hopes to help others not to have to go through what we did to find solutions. You won't have to wonder if only you would have caught it earlier or done things differently. Also, you will be able to answer what can I do while my parent is alive even though they are not physically with me to make life more enjoyable.

There are ways to keep up with your family member's needs when they are far away to ensure their quality of life is the best it can be. We can make those accountable to help us, and it does not have to be difficult.

This book will help you both to meet challenges and encourage you to seek some of your own solutions.

I

Doctors

This is an important chapter as doctors many times can be our greatest hope and sometimes our demise.

Each individual is unique, and all are not made to think or react the same. It is always good to get a second opinion when you feel the answers you have been given do not sit well with you.

There will be doctors that will take the time to ask you questions that others haven't to seek a solution. Some doctors will be able to extend the life of their patients by the extra care, compassion, and taking the time to listen. These doctors are priceless, and I am blessed to know a few.

Unfortunately, there are those doctors that you will be a number, dollar sign, and are not open to listening to their patients. I have also run across doctors with my mother, which helped in her digression until we found a couple of doctors that took time to make a difference. We will be forever thankful to those doctors.

It would help if you asked questions when seeking a doctor for yourself or are becoming a caregiver. When you are a caregiver, your voice is heard to help those who cannot speak for themselves.

Please remember that this book is inspired by those walking in your shoes to help make your days brighter when helping a loved one. When you know you have asked the right questions, gotten answers extended life, and made someone smile, and the whole world looks brighter. The next page is a good step forward.

Questions To Ask

There are questions that need to be asked when seeking a doctor for yourself and especially for a loved one.

1. Were you referred to this physician?

2. Is this physician at a state funded facility? If so, what is the years of experience of this physician?

3. Did they take the time to ask you what your concerns are and if you or your loved one are on any medications?

4. Did they look to see if there were any adverse reactions between the medications that could be causing what you are to see the doctor for?

5. What are the symptoms of having too much of a medication?

6. What are the steps to decrease a medication that is too much and what documentation do you need to get to support the change?

7. Ask them about as the patient gets older whether there can be a decrease in medication. Our systems change as we get older, and we often don't need as much as we used to. I noticed a significant improvement as my mother's prescriptions were minimized to what she needed now. It was not until my mother fell, fractured her spine, and ended up in the hospital that a wonderful doctor looked at her medications. He ended many and decreased others. Why didn't the other doctors look as he did instead of saying she was fine?

8.   Is there a test to see what prescriptions are compatible with your system?

9.   What can or cannot happen by a doctor adding more then one medication to work together? Can they? Are there any possible side effects?

10.   What are the steps to decreasing a medication if needed and how long does it take before you see results?

11.   Is there anything that can be done as far as diet to help?

12.   If weight loss is a problem, are there any shakes that can be added to each meal or in between times?

13.   Can medication be changed to help with appetite? Are there any side affects?

14.   If the person is overweight what can be done with diet to help the person lose excess weight and decrease medications over time?

15.   Can depression medication be decreased over time? Does medication need to be changed from time to time? Can it be lessened? Or does medication need to be increased?

These are just some of the questions that we need to ask to ensure that our loved ones are getting the best care. It is always good not to take it for granted that everything is perfect. We can hope, and sometimes it is perfect. If you check and everything is, then it is validation. If it is not, you know that changes need to be made in one or more areas.

Sugar and Salt

This topic can either make or break your relationship with the facility, staff, and doctor.

There is a time for sugar and not salt, but it is sometimes not always easy to know which time it is.

We must remember that everyone has a life outside of the jobs each of us work that may or may not affect how we react.

It is important to have your facts in order and back them up when you are the one questioning what may need to be changed. Or you may have questions about why certain things have not been done or kept up with.

Generally, you get more done with a good attitude and not a demeanor of hostility. An attitude of understanding helps both parties to find a resolution easier than seeking insults.

A bit of sugar always helps soften the saltiness of a not-so-nice situation. Seek to remember the good things and focus on them, which will help when broaching a topic that is not pleasant.

If you have to be salty to get their attention, then make sure you have your facts.

Remember if you look for problems you will always find them but the same goes for looking for positives. When one door closes another door will open.

Documentation

Documentation is key to being able to show a history of medical, places you have lived, and much more.

Medically you can use documentation to show a list of medications over a period of time, tests taken, test results, and any prior conditions.

When my mother had a doctor lessen and cancel most of her prescriptions when she fell and fractured her spine, it was a wake-up call. A wonderful doctor did what many had not thought to do: look at her medications and see if there might be a reason for falling besides the actual fall.

This doctor made changes that benefited my mother but did not decrease her depression meds. I have noticed that depression medications generally get decreased or changed by the prescribing physician or the doctor who is now in charge. The doctor in charge was new to taking and being her physician.

I will forever be grateful to the doctor for getting the ball rolling to making effective changes for my mother. It brought it to my attention that change was needed. When my mother still had problems with her moods and memory, I looked to see what had not been changed. Her depression medication was not changed at all, and my mother had decreased appetite, memory loss, and other symptoms.

This led me to look up her depression medication to see what the benefits were, the adverse effects of having too much, interaction with other prescriptions, and not having enough. My mother had all the symptoms of having too much.

The symptoms of too much medication resulted in loss of appetite, confusion, and memory loss.

When I discovered this I knew that I could not just ask to have the doctor decrease her depression medication. I also looked up the process for decreasing medication so that I would be informed when I broached the subject to the doctor.

I decided the next step of action was to do more research of what I had learned so that I had more then one source for my argument to help my mother.

When I had several more sources I typed up a letter for additional documentation and explained in detail what I had learned. I also attached the documentation to my letter for the doctor to peruse and make a decision.

Since I had done my due diligence the doctor agreed to decrease my mothers depression medication in increments.

It was amazing to see my mother's mood changed for the better, her appetite increase, and her memory come back. She still has the beginning of dementia, but she no longer asked me when the ship would dock.

There is a lot of importance of properly keeping documentation by writing letters, keeping documents, writing down dates and times when speaking to staff members and doctors. Keeping documentation is instrumental in helping yourself and your loved ones.

Tests

Tests are important as a preventative measure used by doctors to check out whether we have deficiencies, cholesterol, thyroid, and many other medical issues that concern us.

There are a few tests that I believe are important for all of us to take into consideration whether for ourselves or our loved ones.

The following are recommended tests:

<u>GeneSight</u>- this test takes just a swab of the cheek for dna testing that will be used to see how your body metabolizes or responds to different medications. It can be helpful to avoid adverse or allergic reactions. Also, let you know what medications will work together.

<u>Vitamin & Mineral</u>: Vitamin and Mineral deficiencies can lead to life-threatening disease and infection. Many times catching these deficiencies can bring about great results. A blood test is the quickest way to find out. My other book, "Vitamins, Minerals, and More!" does a breakdown of foods, functions of the body, and deficiencies (symptoms). This is a guide to incorporate what foods you may be deficient in into your daily diet. Always consult with a physician you trust.

<u>Hormone</u>: Hormonal tests can explain a lot about our moods, weight gain, and our ability to metabolize. Also, it can affect how we get a good night's sleep.

<u>Stress and Fatigue:</u> Stress and Fatigue can lead to life threatening conditions such as adrenal failure. One of the best advice I have been given was from my doctor who told me I needed to change my life and priorities. She told me to eliminate my stress and when I did it changed my life for the better.

Thyroid- There are two types of thyroid. Hypothyroid is an underactive thyroid that can lead to being overweight, sleep problems, and other problems. Hyperthyroidism can lead to bulging eyes, fast heart rate, weight loss, and abnormal sleep among other problems. Proper medication and diet can make a big difference.

Heart- A heart test can let you know whether or not you have clogged arteries, inflammation, lipids, and other possible abnormalities. It can also let you know if you are doing everything right.

Digestive- deals with the how we process, transport, and transform our food. You can find out if you have a gluten intolerance, liver, kidney, colon, and other possible possible problems. Sometimes diet change can make a world of difference.

     These tests are great preventives to helping yourself or a loved one. Always seek a second opinion if you feel it isn't lining up with how you feel. Also, a good naturopathic doctor can sometimes offer an alternative view and sometimes even more detail. It was a naturopathic doctor that helped me with my thyroid and got me evened out. I have both a naturopathic doctor and a regular physician that I see.

Eyes Open

It is good to have your eyes open, whether you are at home and have helpers, have your loved one in an expensive care home, or a state-funded facility.

When I state your eyes should be wide open, it is because lapses of care can occur even under the best circumstances. It can be as simple as the changing from day to night staff, a new trainee, and just because they may not think it is as important as you do.

How can you manage the simple things that are important to you for your loved one? Of knowing that your loved one has their television on for mental stimulation, not dressed in a hospital gown when you have nice bedtime clothes for them and that they do not leave your loved one in their bed all day instead of taking them to interact with others at mealtime?

You have to make an effort to stop by weekly and sometimes do a surprise visit. If you cannot stop by easily, I would do a video call where you can see how your loved one is and ask the caregiver to show you where they are at. This way, you can see if the television is on, whether your loved one is wearing a hospital gown instead of the gown you purchased for them, and where they are at when you are calling. Are they in their room instead of the cafeteria? Are they in a hospital gown instead of the nice gown you purchased for them? Is the television on or off? These are simple but important matters when you have a loved one that is declining. You want them to be as comfortable, cognitive, and happy as they can be.

Simple solutions to these problems are alerting the nurses and staff heads to these changes that need to be made. I would suggest both calling and putting in writing the changes that need to be made.

It is also good to document each occurrence of the television not being on, hospital gown worn, and when they are not sitting in the cafeteria. This way, you have dates and times that you can use for documentation. It is much easier for them to take you more seriously when you are keeping track.

There are other easy solutions to make your loved one's life nicer by being observant. An example of this is that I noticed each time I scheduled a visit with my mother they would comb her hair and put makeup on her. This happened whether I was on a video call or in person. When I show up unannounced she doesn't have makeup. Makeup makes my mother feel pretty, so now I know what to do to brighten my mother's day. Find out what you can do by being observant and make a day brighter.

I had these problems that reoccurred on a semi-frequent basis that I have had to address with as much sugar and less salt as possible. It was a wonderful nurse that printed up fliers that went above my mother's bed that said the following:

- Please put ******* clothes in her personal closet and not mix in with her roommates.
- Please put *******evening gowns on instead of a hospital gown per her daughter's request as she bought them for her.
- Please put the television on Turner Classics Channel 360 as this is what her daughter requests
- Please take ********down to the cafeteria for lunch and dinner per her daughter's request so she can socialize

I went through a couple of frustrating years asking for solutions before a simple solution was performed. An enclosed closet was a solution brought about by one of the heads of staff. It was amazing how much this simplified matters of other people's clothes mixed in with my mother's and vice-versa.

If your loved one is a man in a facility when you call, they may ensure he is shaved and hair combed. It could be that they also take the time to put a nice shirt on that is in his closet and dress him. A lot of this also depends upon the level of cognition a person has.

I have seen various people in different stages in the nursing home, assisted living, and in-home care. Some are still reading but cannot walk, walk but not remember, and those that simple kindness brighten their day.

We can still make a day brighter by taking action and being observant of their individual needs. When we can figure out what makes a person happy, life is better for the individual and the caregiver.

Whether your loved one is at home or in a facility, keeping your eyes open is important to document to ensure they get the best care possible and consistently.

Another thing to remember is that many people do care. We must be observant of those who your loved one is happy to see. When you see the flaws, it is also essential to see the many positives. It is never too late to give a compliment or an acknowledgment that their kindness has been noticed.

Your situation may be different but seeking solutions is where we all find common ground.

Communication

Communication is key in letting a loved one know that they are cared for and let other family and friends who care keep in contact. This is a blessing to your loved one and the caregiver as they will give you the much-needed support as your loved one continues to decline.

Today's technology enables us to video chat and also add people to these chats. I, personally, would rather call each family member or close friend so that they can enjoy the one-on-one familiarity.

Sending flowers, cards, and letters also are a great way to brighten an otherwise daily routine to show the love. You or the caregiver can read the letter or card to them making it a special time.

When you make it a weekly call to a loved one or stop by, it helps brighten their day and also helps to decrease their decline. They have something to look forward to while they see others who do not, unfortunately.

My family has been very supportive since I became the one in charge of my mother's welfare. They are supportive because I keep them all in the loop of what is going on, calls I have made, letters sent, and the documentation to back it up. They feel better knowing my mother is being looked after correctly, and their supportiveness makes my job that much easier. It is not easy being the one to be the warden to ensure things are being done. It does not make me happy to tell others what they are lacking, but my mother's welfare is at stake.

Communication is key in all things and with as much sugar as possible without a lot of salt.

Stages

When my father died my mother decided she did not have to take care of herself anymore. Initially, we did not know as she kept herself busy with family and friends.

Later, one of my family members found different pills on the floor in various locations and this was just the beginning of a downward decline.

The doctors at that time did not do my mother any favors and now I see she was just another number and dollar sign.

There are many good doctors and there are those who just go through the motions. We are brought up to trust in the process and believe they care enough to do right by our loved ones. I believe that there is a possibility that earlier awareness of my mother's medications prescribed by her doctors of the side effects would have been a clue. God turns all things around for the good so am hoping this is being used for that purpose.

So here are some of the following stages that you may need to be aware of and not necessarily in this exact order:

- Finding pills on the floor
- Walking slower
- Unable to walk long distances
- Needing to stop more frequently
- Unable to stand for long distances
- Memory declines
- Double dosing
- Not wanting to shower
- Not wanting to get hair washed
- Not picking up after themselves
- Not able to work a phone

- Taste changes - example no longer liking sweets
- Loss of appetite
- Incontinent
- Falling
- Sleeping more
- Unable to do simple tasks
- Voice lowers in level and is harder to hear
- Repeating themselves
- Asking questions again and again
- Looking to you for validation
- Combative verbally
- Combative physically
- No longer able to work a television
- No longer available to work a computer

These are just some of the stages to be aware of that may help you to be able to proactive in helping your loved one sooner.

Sometimes we get so involved in our own lives that we do not see what is in front of us.

Let this list be a good start in being proactive in your loved ones life.

Home Care

This chapter is dedicated to giving you a heads up on some of the things that you will need for caring for your loved one.

Here are some of the following that you will need and not necessarily in this order:

1. Hand bars for the bathroom
2. Hand bars for the shower
3. A shower chair
4. Baby shampoo
5. Sanitary wipes
6. Wheel chair accessible
7. Dry shampoo
8. List of doctors
9. List of medications
10. Insurance cards and phone numbers
11. Baby monitor
12. Inside cameras
13. List of family members phone numbers
14. Family Trust
15. Durable Power Of Attorney
16. Medical Power Of Attorney

This is just a start, but at least this is a good beginning list to help.

Your List

22

www.ingramcontent.com/pod-product-compliance
Lightning Source LLC
Chambersburg PA
CBHW070847220526
45466CB00002B/906